One Man's Perspective:

Venesa Strong's Journey through Dementia

Lester M. Strong, Caregiver, Spouse
Commentary: Robert D. Harbaugh, M.D.
Edited: Karen Aldenderfer

NOTICE: This book provides information about the progression of Lewy body dementia particular to Venesa Strong. Her experiences are not necessarily typical of the disease, as Venesa did not experience many of the hallmark features of LBD. It should not be considered to be medical advice or as a guide to diagnosis and treatment of the disease. Guidance must come only from consultation with a qualified physician. The author disclaims any liability in connection with the use of this information.

Review of medical information: Robert Harbaugh, M.D.
Editing, cover and book design, and book layout: Karen Aldenderfer
Printed by CreateSpace, an Amazon.com company
Available online from CreateSpace.com and Amazon.com
ISBN-13: 9781976513015
ISBN-10: 19766513014

Dedicated to Venesa,
the love of my life and lifelong partner

Table of Contents

Venesa Strong's Journey—Introduction	5
What is Lewy Body Disease? The Short Story	8
Identifying the Symptoms of the Subset of LBD Maladies Venesa Had	11
Meet Venesa	13
Early Presentation of Symptoms— Mild Cognitive Impairment	19
Moderate (Middle Stage) Lewy Body Dementia	27
Diagnosis: Lewy Body Dementia	29
Setting General Ground Rules for the Future	33
My Struggles as a Homemaker	36
Coping with Loneliness and Depression	42
Coping with the Progression of LBD Dementia	45
Nothing is Impossible—Journeying with Dementia	51
Maintaining Skills in the Face of Decline	62
Choosing Caregiver Support	65
Ongoing Adaptations in the Face of Ongoing Decline	68
Approaching Venesa's Final Days	79
Venesa's Legacy	82

Venesa Strong's Journey
Introduction

This short book was written to succinctly provide a broad overview of Venesa's path through Lewy body disease (LBD) from the initial indications years before her formal diagnosis through her final days. The methods, techniques, risks, and activities used by her husband and caregiver to keep Venesa happy, active, comfortable, and enjoying life are clearly articulated with an explanation of the associated rationale of each. The focus of this narrative is from a male caregiver's perspective (her spouse, Lester Strong). The information contained provides "just the right" amount of information for (a) the newly diagnosed patient and his/her family; (b) distant family members, friends, or close associates who need the essential profile of this disorder without having to resort to sources with "too much information"; and (c) as a reference text.

    A more complete book on LBD by Dr. Robert D. Harbaugh, MD, is expected in early 2018, to take the understanding of this disease to the next level for the lay public. High-level, easy-to-understand medical insight will be provided, as well as a full description of LBD characteristics, many of which were not manifest in Venesa's case. There are several other excellent lay oriented, more in-depth books available, with more exhaustive reference texts specifically written for non-professionals that should complement the above referenced book and this narrative. Should the reader be a principal caregiver, he/she should create a library of references. The more one knows about a complex medical disorder, the better that person—whether as the affected one or the caregiver—will do. This book attempts to provide simplicity and succinctness, perhaps as the "first read" on the subject, employing sufficient breadth to allow the reader to see the bigger picture of this complex disorder.

Lester Strong spent 24 hours per day seven days a week for approximately eight years caring for his wife, Venesa, who was formally diagnosed with Lewy body dementia May 13, 2011. However, it was evident that the disease had started much earlier. She passed March 12, 2016.

Strong, author of this book, is an electrical engineer, not a physician, and it is his hands-on experience—along with many discussions, emails and doctor appointments with Venesa's primary care physician and two neurologists—that provide the "authority" of the information presented in this book. Although this disease had a tremendous impact on Les' life and impacted his children's lives, this is not the point of the manuscript.

Robert Harbaugh—a neurologist, with more than 30 years' experience in late-life neurodegenerative disorders—provided care for Venesa in her later years. After Venesa's passing, Strong approached Dr. Harbaugh with a request for commentary in this manuscript, feeling that their experiences and very different perspectives would complement each other.

One of the significant lessons I learned is that there is no replacement for a complete and open relationship with the physicians. Venesa and I enjoyed many activities that I might not have attempted had I not been encouraged by her physicians first. There was risk involved and a risk/reward decision to be made. Virtually every time the physicians made accommodations to minimize the risk and, after discussion with us, recommended we, "go for it." Venesa was ecstatic because these were the things she truly loved or made her very happy. Every activity worked out well!

The author hopes this attempt to provide a compelling narrative to explain Venesa's LBD issues and Les' caregiver techniques will benefit patients, their families, and caregivers. Those wanting to learn more about complex medical disorders, whether with a lay or professional background, should utilize several information sources and always apply critical thinking when presented with novel approaches or breakthrough method of intervention. As some say, "In God we trust; in everyone else we validate."

Lester Strong
Robert Harbaugh

What is Lewy Body Disease?
The Short Story

Dementia, in essence, refers to an acquired disorder of the central nervous that creates a generally progressive loss of independent living. Dementia creates variable degrees of impaired cognitive abilities among a variety of spheres, and often yields changes in personality and behavior. Dementia is not a specific disease, but a syndrome created by one or more specific underlying brain disorders. Thus, dementia is an umbrella term much like the term cancer. There are many types of cancer such as breast, lung, bladder, prostate or ovarian cancer. Dementia includes multiple neurological degenerative diseases such as Lewy body dementia (LBD), Parkinson's disease, Alzheimer's disease, frontotemporal dementia, vascular dementia, among others. LBD was not well known to specialists until the late 1990s! The reasons for this are complex and are in part due to the inability to accurately identify Lewy bodies in parts of the brain until the last two decades of the 20th century. Only in the past few years have physicians become familiar with this disorder. LBD conservatively affects 2.5–3 million Americans at this time and is the second most common type of progressive dementia after Alzheimer's.

    LBD is caused by abnormal clusters of protein deposits called Lewy bodies in the cells within areas of the brain disrupting memory and movement. *Tau* proteins may also be present surrounding Lewy bodies causing neurofibrillary tangles resulting in communication difficulties between cells. Commonly, beta amyloid plaques, a hallmark of Alzheimer's disease, are seen microscopically in people with LBD.

    Typically, LBD affects each individual with only a subset of the broad spectrum of the possible maladies that define the disease. The symptoms Venesa exhibited included deficits in attention, memory function, autonomic dysfunction, significant mobility difficulties, cognitive impairment, hallucinations, speech difficulties, difficulty eating, hyposmia (inability to detect odors), lack of bladder and bowel control, and increased need for sleep throughout the day. She experienced a few falls, fainting, depression, anxiety, delusions, and hallucinations; she was always pleasant and cooperative, never wandered (although, for safety reasons, the house was set up to prevent that) and she typically slept peacefully through the night. Venesa' enthusiasm for travel and outings provided continuous stimulation. Despite the disease, she remained the kind and thoughtful person she had always been. On the other hand, Venesa never experienced some of the other hallmark symptoms of the disease, such as sundowning, combative behavior, or exhibited REM sleep disorder, which will be fully covered in the 2018 book on LBD. This book is intended to be a case study of Venesa and her experiences with the subset of LBD maladies she dealt with.

    Currently there are no available techniques to quantitatively diagnose LBD as there is no imaging technique sufficiently sensitive to see the protein in the brain—the only way to positively identify the presence of Lewy bodies is to perform a biopsy with thin slices of the brain under a high power microscope. Interesting to note that the medical community is on the verge of associating "biomarkers" (quantitative measures, such as specific molecules highly associated with one type of dementia and not others) in everyday medical practice; currently, such biomarkers are benefiting from rapid deployment in research settings. However, at the time of this writing, there are no widely available, applicable biomarkers that have high utility in LBD. Nonetheless, stay tuned!

    Venesa's diagnosis was done with circumstantial evidence using data and expert opinion gathered by a group of expert medical personnel from several disciplines. A medical assessment and verbal and written testing suggested that the most likely diagnosis was LBD.

While there are currently no disease-modifying interventions for LBD, the wealth of strategies—including the cautious use of certain medications coupled with caregiver education and commitment—can greatly improve quality of life for those affected by the disease.

Identifying the Symptoms
of the Subset of LBD Maladies Venesa Had

As described earlier, LBD, one of the dementia diseases, is characterized by progressive cognitive impairment that eventually precludes a person's independent function. The earliest symptoms/signs Venesa encountered were memory problems, visuospatial deficits, and cognitive impairments, problem solving difficulties, language deficits, and personality changes.

Cognitive highs and lows (sometimes referred to as Fluctuations) in cognition will be noticeable to those who are close to the person with LBD, such as coworkers, partners, and relatives. At times, the person will be alert and then suddenly have acute episodes of confusion and/or inattention. These may last minutes, hours, or days! Fluctuations are not related to delirium, sundowning, or pathological sleepiness, but may overlap and be indistinguishable. While other dementias may also display fluctuations, it is not to the extent and severity as those with LBD. However, not all LBD patients display easily identifiable fluctuations.

Hallucinations (false sensory perceptions) are predominantly visual and tend to be more pronounced when the person is most confused. They are not necessarily frightening to the person, but are associated with heightened anxiety. Other modalities of hallucinations rarely observed involve sound, taste, smell, and touch. Certain medications can exacerbate the frequency of hallucinations, but do not cause the appearance of hallucinations.

Parkinsonism (Parkinson's disease symptoms), takes the form of changes in gait, speed of movement, stiffness and, occasionally, tremor. The person will typically shuffle or walk stiffly, either symmetrically or asymmetrically. There may also be frequent unexplained falls. Blank stares, emotionless facial expressions are observed, as well as a stooped posture and, with progression of the disease, drooling may be present. Venesa did not have symptoms of Parkinsonism until halfway through the process.

Visuospatial difficulties, including impairments in depth perception, object orientation, directional sense, and illusions may occur.

Autonomic dysfunction, is now recognized as a cardinal feature of LBD, and may include blood pressure fluctuations, heart rate variability, sexual disturbances/impotence, constipation(rarely diarrhea), urinary problems (most often incontinence), excessive sweating or decreased sweating/heat intolerance, fainting, dry eyes/mouth, and complex changes in oropharyngeal function (e.g., increased salivation and drooling, and difficulty swallowing).

Robert D. Harbaugh, MD

Meet Venesa

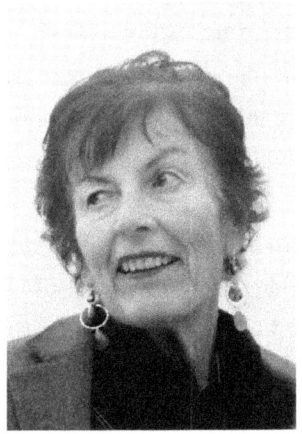

Venesa's Favorite Prayer—
Peace Prayer of Saint Francis

Lord, make me an instrument of your peace. Where there is hatred, let me sow love; where there is injury, pardon; where there is doubt, faith; where there is despair, hope; where there is darkness, light; and where there is sadness, joy.

Divine Master, grant that I may not so much seek to be consoled as to console; to be understood as to understand; to be loved as to love; for it is in giving that we receive; it is in pardoning that we are pardoned; and that it is in dying that we are born to eternal life.

Attributed to St. Francis of Assisi

Venesa W. Strong

Venesa . . . Venesa Strong. Aptly named. This story is about an incredible strong woman. A woman who was a devoted wife and mother. A woman who was passionate about her work and her family. A woman who was active and adventurous and "game for anything."

    Venesa was born at West Lafayette, Indiana, in 1941 just as her father followed his sense of responsibility to support the country and enlisted in the army. For the first six years of Venesa's life she lived in a single-parent household with her mother spending a lot of time with Venesa'a grandparents, Mammaw and Papa. Papa had a great influence on her development. He was quiet, sweet, and had a fun loving manner. Venesa told me that Papa would trail behind her wherever she chose to go at her speed. When her father, a major in the Army, returned from service he tried to run the house as orderly as he managed his troops (very unlike Papa). He returned to a strong-willed six-year-old daughter who hardly knew him. Obviously, conflict ensued between Venesa and her father, not unmanageable but it made life difficult—her father's absence had resulted in his having little influence on her early development. Her mother, however, was the strongest influence in Venesa's development. Soon after her father returned from the service, Venesa's sister, Sally, was born and three years later her brother, Howard, was born.

    Venesa's father, Richard, took a job in Cleveland, Ohio, in tractor sales, until an opportunity for promotion arose and the family moved to Michigan. There Richard was able to achieve his dream—they bought a farm and he became a "gentleman farmer" while continuing to work his sales job. This, however, did not last long; an even greater opportunity presented itself and the family moved to Alhambra, CA in the Los Angeles area, then Stockton and Lodi, selling steel buildings. Although Richard was successfully climbing the corporate ladder in sales, he decided to venture out on his own when the next opportunity came up that would require him to move his family. By then, Venesa was in high school. Richard's self-employment became a financial burden the family was not accustomed to. Venesa'a mother took a job to help with the family finances. Beginning at the age of 12, Venesa was responsible for the creation of menus, shopping for food, and preparing the family dinners within a budget. This really helped when both her parents went to work. Since Lodi was so very hot in the summer, Venesa would do her chores in the morning, spend the afternoon at the local pool, and return to the final stages of dinner at the last minute. The heat also drove Venesa and her father to the local public tennis court at 5:00 a.m. to play tennis.

    When Venesa graduated from high school her father requested that she defer college for a year and attend a secretarial school to provide her with useful skills to work her way through college if that became necessary. Venesa had to "help out" by earning and paying 20% of her undergraduate college education in any case. Once in secretarial school, Venesa felt like a fish out of water—her peers seemed to be husband shopping and could not comprehend Venesa's determination to get through her studies. Freshman year at the Oregon State University, Venesa pledged the Kappa Alpha Theta sorority. She was devastated when her mother was unable to attend the sorority's Mother's Day celebration due to financial constraints. Richard was not as successful an entrepreneur as he had been as a corporate salesman. Upon graduating with a Bachelor of Science in Home Economics, majoring in nutrition, Venesa was immediately off to Massachusetts General Hospital (Harvard) as an intern toward the formal Registered Dietitian Certification, which she completed. She then took a job in Houston, Texas, as a Registered Dietitian managing the kitchen service. There she was surprised to find that two of her best friends at Massachusetts General had been hired at the same hospital. The three women roomed together for several years and remained best friends throughout Venesa's demise.

After a few years in Texas, Venesa decided to increase her education and she enrolled at Cornell University in Ithaca, New York, where she received the degree of Master's of Nutritional Science and met Lester Strong, who later became her husband. Lester, a PhD candidate in engineering, saw a beautiful lady (Venesa) sitting alone in the graduate dining room. He asked if he could join her, she consented, but before he could set his tray down, Venesa picked up her tray and abruptly said "I am done" and left. That evening, however, they saw each other again in the downstairs coffee shop during a coffee break and they ended up sipping coffee together and enjoyed each other's company for hours.

Lester returned to work at Eastman Kodak in Rochester, New York, yet continued to date Venesa although she was still at Cornell. Once Venesa graduated, she took a job at the Visiting Nurse Service in Rochester, and after several years in Rochester they decided to get married. They were blessed with their first child in Rochester, Jeffrey Nelson, in 1974. In the mid-1970s Venesa announced that she had not realized when they married that she would have to live in the city of her husband's choice, and that they needed to look for a job in California. Lester had never been west of the Mississippi, however, he found employment at Vandenberg Air Force Base. Venesa took a part-time position teaching at California Polytechnic University (Cal Poly).

While shopping for a house in Santa Maria they joined the local country club to have access to the tennis courts and to meet people in the community. Venesa's love for tennis led her to take lessons and graduate from Vic Braden Tennis College in 1978. While in Santa Maria, they were blessed with a second son, Richard "Chad" Chadwick in 1979.

Venesa was instrumental in keeping both boys active in their chosen sports. Jeff enjoyed tennis and was given local lessons from a very young age, graduating to higher level classes out of town. While in junior high school Jeff played men's open in Los Angeles and in high school he obtained a tennis scholarship in the Pac 10. Chad played baseball locally in high school, the local summer collegiate baseball team, the traveling team from Carson California and in college for the Miami Hurricanes where he won the College World Series.

Cal Poly as not challenging enough for Venesa, so she began to consult on nutrition in local industry while still teaching at Cal Poly. In her ongoing quest for knowledge, in the late 1990s Venesa decided to get an executive Master's Degree in business from the University of California, Los Angeles. She commuted from Santa Maria several hundred miles each way to achieve this. Venesa loved to travel; she represented the State Department in Cuba, and took a second State Department trip to China when it first opened to the Western world. She spent three months in India, several months in Mexico for immersion in Spanish, traveling to Peru for the International Congress of Dietetics and visited Machu Picchu (Peru) while she was there. Venesa also visited Russia and, of course, took in the traditional sights of Europe.

Venesa was hit with a horrible disease in 2002, Lewy body dementia. It robbed her of her memory and held her prisoner in her own body—ultimately unable to talk, eat, walk, or take care of her own personal needs. This is the unfolding story of how we lived, traveled, coped, and persevered throughout the course of this devastating disease. Venesa had the gift to be able to live one day at a time, facing each challenge as it arose, and doing whatever was required. She never realized that she had LBD and we never talked about it.

Progression of Venesa's Lewy Body Dementia

Mild Cognitive Impairment (MCI), 2002–2008
Early Stage Lewy Body Dementia, 2008–mid 2010
Moderate Middle Stage Lewy Body Dementia, mid 2010–mid 2013
Severe Late Stage Lewy Body Dementia, mid 2013–2016

Early Presentation of Symptoms—
Mild Cognitive Impairment

In 2002, years before Venesa was formally diagnosed with LBD, very subtle changes began to occur that were clearly out of character for her but not of significant magnitude to cause serious concern. Because the changes were so gradual, these incidents were easy to overlook or excuse. In retrospect, however, the frequency of these minor incidents, their timeline, and their integrated impact were considerable.

As is often the case for family members, I gave it little importance until my brother and his wife met us at the Pasadena New Year's Parade in 2008. They pointed out to me that Venesa's actions, her memory, and conversational ability had clearly deteriorated.

Perhaps because they had not seen Venesa for some time, they recognized the severity of the deterioration in her behavior. My brother called me after returning home and told me that they knew what was happening and, suspecting dementia, he warned me that I was going to have to learn to live without Venesa. They had noticed significant changes in her memory. Her conversation was not as it used to be, and intellectually she was not the same. And sure enough, having retired, I was so close to Venesa— virtually 24 hours each day—that I had not perceived this very slow and subtle deterioration in her cognitive skills. With fierce denial, I initially rationalized that they had not seen her for so long that they were not really remembering things properly and I disregarded their comments. There is such safety in denial!

But a second incident occurred in late 2009. While working as a consultant for a client for whom she had worked for years, Venesa inadvertently removed a patient's very confidential file from a work facility, forgetting she had put it into her briefcase when she left. Clearly, this breached protocol and it was returned as soon as noticed. Fortunately, there were no repercussions or other actions taken, but it was imperative that Venesa immediately leave that client. At this time I had no idea that Venesa was suffering from anything, much less that she was in the early stages of LBD. However, in retrospect, it underscores the imprudence of conducting business while afflicted with MCI or LBD—particularly one with sensitive tasks that require critical thinking. I am sure Venesa would never have done this had she not been in the initial stages of dementia. But at the time, I ignored it as a reasonable mistake.

Not long afterward, as part of our tasks as voluntary ushers for the local Junior College Performing Arts Theater, Venesa became confused handing out programs and ushering people to their seats. She was clearly not able to perform the task and I realized this would be our last performance as ushers.

During this period, I would run very short errands to pick up a few items at the grocery store, leaving Venesa at home. Once after a short 15-minute errand, the moment Venesa heard the garage door open she raced to the door leading into the house with a wonderful smile on her face. She exclaimed, "You did come home!" and gave me a big hug in relief. This spontaneous gesture was the only time she demonstrated her fear of being abandoned! I was so fortunate that she had not left the house and wandered off trying to find me!

To some extent, the hallmarks of LBD were masked by Venesa's significant difficulty in walking caused by her defective knees. She had had arthroscopic knee surgery in April 1989 yet had continued to have knee problems until it culminated in January 2010, when she had a partial replacement of her right knee. Despite surgery, this led to 14 months of agony; the components of her knee immediately shifted, causing significant pain. A total replacement of her right knee was done in February 2011 followed by a total replacement of her left knee in August. After rehabilitation, both replacements were a total success in the end.

However, there were three issues with the knee replacements:

(1) Foremost, the complexities of surgery, medications, and rehabilitation from knee replacement surgery masked Venesa's encroaching dementia. At the time, I attributed her pain, behavior, and lack of cognition to the knee replacement and did not even consider a potential developing cognitive issue.

(2) Both of the first two surgeries used extremely potent narcotic drugs. The narcotics for the first surgery caused what I considered very scary behavior during recovery, including hallucinations, lack of responsiveness, difficulty in communicating, and an apparent lack of understanding. Venesa's reaction after her second surgery were even stronger, exhibiting the same characteristics during recovery and culminating with her curling up in a corner of the room in fetal position with her hands clasped and playing with her fingers. I was beside myself, thinking I had lost her then. This was the first time I experienced a situation that was so closely aligned to the horror psychological movies of experimental facilities from the 1950s. They had never been pleasant to watch on film, and I clearly did not like to experience it firsthand with my loved one! When I addressed the situation with the doctor and medical staff, I was told that the OxyContin would just wear off and all would be well. However, Venesa's hallucinations and her lack of cognition and understanding persisted, while her inability to recognize people was intermittent. I blamed this on the anesthesia, still without

thinking of the possibility of dementia. In retrospect, I wonder if these narcotics had triggered or perhaps accelerated her dementia. For the third surgery, I did not let the doctor use any narcotics; the surgery went flawlessly without them, Venesa did not experience any adverse effects from the surgery, and both the doctor and I were elated.

(3) Despite having a good reputation, the doctor that had done Venesa's first surgery was careless in procedure and superficial in treatment, yet demanding in payment and unwilling to take Medicare. In realizing this, I found a new doctor that did take Medicare. The new doctor had been performing approximately 8 to 12 knee replacements every Monday, Wednesday, and Friday for quite some time. He was a thoughtful, careful doctor and performed a successful surgery with no side effects and very satisfactory results. Oh how I wished I had found him first, but this underscores the importance getting a second opinion, and researching the doctor and the procedures prior to surgery. Hindsight and experience are always so instructive!

Another reality check was in January 2011 when our eldest son, Jeff, was married. We made trips to Los Angeles to shop for a mother-of-the-groom dress and accessories with little issue. However, leading up to and during the wedding Venesa exhibited cognitive, physical, and mobility issues similar to those we had blamed on her partial knee replacement a year earlier. About two months before the wedding, she began to experience difficulties in mobility, which became more exaggerated as time progressed and were clearly noticeable at the reception. She could only wear the beautiful formal gown she had chosen for about ten minutes before she had to change to something that gave her greater freedom and would allow her easier movement and increased comfort.

Further, Venesa exhibited significant cognitive impairment; her sister, Sally, was devastated when Venesa did not recognize her that day, although with time, the recognition eventually returned. While Venesa was able to dance with the groom, it took a great deal of effort on her part. In retrospect, I think that there was much more brewing than simply knee problems and associated pain, possibly announcing to us the encroachment of dementia.

Most alarming was the realization that Venesa had lost her postural reflexes. Walking with her friends in early 2011, Venesa tripped over a slight irregularity in the concrete. Having no reaction to try and catch herself, break her fall, or recover in any other way, she fell flat on her face breaking a tooth.

Most of Venesa's friends had become frustrated with her as the disease encroached and would no longer come over to visit her. Although they respected her as a brilliant, friendly, and personable individual, they felt that if this could happen to her it could happen to any one of them, and they said they could not face up to that. Others did not know what to say to her. Although I encouraged her friends to visit albeit briefly, none would come and she became increasingly isolated with only brief "hellos" from former friends when I took her to the country club for lunch. Still, Venesa's behavioral changes occurred so slowly and subtly that they were difficult for me to discern and it continued to be easy to overlook or excuse. Quite simply, I continued to blame the knee surgeries and the anesthetics. But as time progressed, Venesa went from having relatively normal mobility and cognition to extremely difficult mobility, reduced cognition, and a sharp increased need for sleep.

Many families/caregivers may have a hard time conveying to others that their loved one really has early mild cognitive impairment during the first few years of clinical manifestations. In the early stage, a person will look "perfectly" OK on cursory contact, particularly if they do not see the person often.

Subtle parkinsonism, mild gait instability, variable forgetfulness, questionable judgment, sporadic spatial disorientation, strange sleep disorders, quirky beliefs (e.g., delusions) and fleeting visual hallucinations can be easily overlooked in the aging adult with "forgetfulness," especially, when the observations are, by nature, inconsistent. Precisely because of the patient's ability to perform remarkably well (appear normal) when put in the spotlight early in the disease, other people may become skeptical of the problem. It is often only a spouse, child, or close confidant who will have enough continuous exposure to clearly appreciate the changes.

Although one's natural inclination is to try to convince disbelieving relatives that there is, indeed, "something wrong"— particularly relatives who don't have constant contact—don't stress over their denial. Keep them updated as the disease progresses, and in time, they will come to see the full force of the manifestations for themselves, once the disease is finally diagnosed as LBD.

Venesa and I went to church in May 2012 and about 20 minutes into the service while standing up and singing a hymn, Venesa said she did not feel well and needed to sit down, so we did. A short time thereafter, during the sermon, she said she really did not feel well. We got up and started to leave. After five or six steps she totally collapsed into my arms and I gently let her down to the floor. It took several church members to help me get her into a church wheelchair and into my car. I took her to the emergency room where she was diagnosed with extremely low blood pressure. The doctor reduced two of her medications. After we made the necessary reductions, things seemed to be much better.

Despite her subtle decline, Venesa continued her membership in a ladies' stock investment club. She had joined the club in early 2010 and remained active in the organization through early 2013—this club being the last remaining social outlet for her. But after three years and a gradual deterioration in gait and cognition, it began to be apparent to the group that something was not right. When Venesa began to sleep through most of the meeting without participating in it, one of the women in the group requested that I have Venesa resign. While I was reluctant to isolate her further, I relented when the woman insisted that the entire group wanted her to quit. I felt that Venesa should not be where she was not wanted and that it would be detrimental to her to remain in that environment, so in 2013 she resigned. With this, I was finally able to recognize the root of the problem: Lewy body dementia. Perhaps I had thought that the progression would be much slower, but by this time, it was probably mid-stage LBD.

During the past two decades, refinements in technologies and diagnostic criteria have determined that subtle nascent symptoms characteristic of the disease and early neuropathological changes reflecting the presence of Lewy bodies may occur up to 10 years (or more) before a clear-cut diagnosis of LBD can confidently be made. Current clinical criteria requires a high level of clinical involvement to be identified and are not particularly sensitive to the subtleties of the disorder. Many with early LBD may be overlooked since they do not manifest sufficient involvement to meet clinical criteria for a label. However, increased public and professional awareness is seeing rising levels of disease knowledge. Despite this, some affected families lament the fact that despite seeking specialty consultations, several years may transpire before a confident diagnosis can be made even when the features of LBD are clearly present.

LBD may progress in a non-linear fashion, with alternating periods of rapid decline, stabilization, unexplained improvements, and further decline—and in some, as Dr. Harbaugh has coined it "the dementia that gets better" (temporarily). On rare occasions, dramatic postoperative or illness-induced (e.g., pneumonia) delirium may be the heralding feature, with subsequent distinct LBD features not expressed for long periods (years in some cases). Alternatively, one may see recurrent periods of psychoses or disabling depressive episodes in late life, often with hospitalizations and, as other LBD features become apparent, eventually leading to a more confident diagnosis.

Moderate (Middle Stage) Lewy Body Dementia
The Path to a Diagnosis

Venesa had been diagnosed with atrial fibrillation years earlier, in 2003. An attempted cardioversion that year had not been successful, and after wearing a ZIO patch for a week to monitor her heart, she required emergency installation of a pacemaker that December. Thereafter cardiac monitoring was required about every six months by Venesa's Stanford cardiologist. By 2010 Venesa's cardiologist commented on the behavioral changes he was observing and he referred us to one of the Stanford neurologists to assess her behavior. An appointment was set up with Dr. Geoffrey A. Kerchner[1]. Dr. Kerchner taught at Stanford University, conducted dementia research four days each week, and saw patients once a week at the Stanford Clinic. After his first assessment, Dr. Kerchner's recommended a follow-up appointment for an in-depth analysis. Having heard that many patients with dementia will often resist a medical evaluation for fear of learning a terrible truth or being stigmatized by the results, I was apprehensive about subjecting Venesa to this complex series of tests, however, the critical need was there, so we agreed. Our second appointment consisted of several days of meetings with his neurological team, including other neurologists, psychiatrists, psychologists, and lab technicians, among others.

    Each medical professional met with Venesa separately, performing oral and written cognitive tests, as well as assessing her balance, mobility, heart, and taking draws for blood tests. Venesa was asked questions to assess her awareness of her

---

[1] MD PhD, Harvard University; Associate Professor of Neurology, Department of Neurology and Neurological Sciences, Stanford Center for Memory Disorders, Stanford University.

current environment, such as what city she was in, the date and time of day, who she was with among other things. Venesa, however, had no apparent reaction to the procedures and there was no indication that she really understood what it meant. During each of the individual tests, Venesa appeared to be relaxed and seemingly enjoyed the interaction with the attending personnel. I was very much relieved by her response. But that in itself could have been an indication of how far advanced she was in the disease by that time. The testing culminated in a team meeting to generate a consensus between examiners, which was relayed to us on a Friday the 13th of May 2011.

Diagnosis: Lewy Body Dementia

Based on overwhelming circumstantial evidence, the medical team agreed that the most likely diagnosis was LBD, cautioning that there is no fine-focused X-ray available that is sufficiently sensitive to observe the Lewy Bodies in the brain to confirm the diagnosis. The only absolute diagnosis would require an autopsy, fine slices of brain tissue, and a very powerful microscope.

Dr. Kerchner notified us that, effective immediately, Venesa was no longer considered competent to drive a car (he was mandated to notify the DMV of Venesa's condition and her license would probably be suspended pending formal complete re-certification). She was also not competent to handle cash or credit cards, as her judgement was impaired. Throughout our entire marriage, whenever Venesa and I were in the car together, I would always drive. It became our tradition (this was also the philosophy of my parents so did not seem unusual to me). We were always together once I retired so Venesa had no need or desire to drive. It was a very natural progression for her to stop driving, so she had not driven a car for months before this testing and diagnosis. We never felt a need to discuss it and I always made it a point to accommodate her needs for transportation, so she never felt stranded. The loss of independence that comes with not driving and is so problematic to many early-stage patients was simply not an issue to her, and the transition was so smooth that I had one less thing to worry about. Venesa had no apparent reaction to the diagnosis and there was no indication that she really understood what it meant. Again, I was very much relieved by her reaction.

Throughout this initial time frame, Venesa was reasonably functional despite occasional lapses in memory and episodes of confusion, she was perfectly capable of having normal conversations and being my usual companion. Occasionally she would have difficulty walking, but her mobility was not seriously compromised.

While we also saw other doctors, Dr. Kerchner followed Venesa and the progression of her LBD for the rest of her life.

Welcome to the roller coaster world of Lewy body disease! Learning about its characteristics explained so much about Venesa's behavior and capabilities.

An early typical sign of LBD is occasional loss of attention and alertness, the "on-off" sign when thinking and memory abilities fade out and the person tends to "zone" out from conversations or activities. Forgetting what one is discussing mid-sentence is sometimes observed. Moments of clear functioning may switch to states of confusion that may affect conversation and activities such as successfully preparing a meal, managing personal care, or walking. One might experience difficulties for a few hours and then return to normal functioning; conversely, the difficulties may last a few hours or days. Family members have described the LBD-related changes in attention and alertness as the person's mind being "someplace else" and the person's face getting a "glazed look." Others have described it as being "unconscious, but awake," or "staring" into space for long periods (daydreaming). When asked about what they were thinking, a vague response or "non-answer" is generally given. Other caregivers will describe the patient as having periods of disorganized speech, followed by the inexplicable return to coherent thinking. Some studies have even shown rapidly changing levels of attention, which in theory might create the appearance of a spell, a seizure or stroke, but is neither.

These fluctuations are one of the most remarkable—yet frustrating—aspects of LBD. They are typically without explanation, clearly exceeding the caregiver's inherent sense of what normal day-

to-day variability should be for that person. Caregivers of patients with LBD have noted that when put in certain situations that may require a higher level of functioning (such as seeing the doctor, interfacing with distant family, etc.) their loved ones may "pull it together" for the occasion and perform well, seemingly freer of fluctuations for a period of time.

Fluctuations may dismay the novice caregiver, who may mistakenly interpret the inexplicable changes in behavior as faking or willful fabrication, perhaps for dramatic effect. However, friends and/or relatives who observe the variable alertness, thinking, or behavior must be made aware of this important manifestation of the disease. The remarkable fluctuations seen in most, but not all people with LBD are the direct result of changes in the brain itself, although they are not completely understood at this time. However, since the types of fluctuations observed in alertness overlap with the ubiquitous presence of the wide variety of sleep disorders seen in LBD, a commonality likely resides in the alerting structures within the brainstem. **Learning this explained so much about Venesa's behavior.**

We were told that the best description of LBD is "Alzheimer's disease coupled with Parkinson's disease, accompanied with hallucinations." In terms of a prognosis, we were told that the disease does not follow a typical sequence of events or a "normal" timeline, as each case is unique and follows its own course and time. In Dr. Harbaugh's experience only about 15% of people with LBD get a proper diagnosis when first seen by a specialist, although this percentage seems to be increasing.

One of the biggest concerns is pinpointing when the disease really began. Diagnosis is normally long after initial onset of the disease once the symptoms are fully recognizable, as we saw in Venesa's case. In actuality, it has probably been developing in its early stages for years, largely imperceptible. Once a patient is diagnosed with LBD, he/she may live an average of about eight years post diagnosis before succumbing to the disease, but, again, that can vary substantially from person to person. It has been said "If you have seen a case of LBD you have seen *only* one case." With its diverse nature, one case is characteristically different from the next—almost unrecognizable.

Our reaction to the diagnosis and intentional focus on the future was to take one day at a time. The future, in terms of Venesa's sustained capability and longevity, was deemed to be uncertain with many bumps in the road. And yet, we did not intend to limit our activities; instead we intended to enjoy life to the fullest despite this wrinkle in our plans. Despite our friends cautioning us to curtail our travels, I countered that Venesa loved to travel and if some set back or demise should occur while we were away, it would at least have happened while she was doing one of her favorite activities. Still, there were adjustments to be made.

Setting General Ground Rules for the Future

Financial planning: As luck would have it, in 2008 and before diagnosis, Venesa and I had gone to an attorney to generate a trust, the Lester & Venesa Strong Trust of January 28, 2009. Several legal documents were generated: the Trust, Community Property Agreements, Nomination of Conservators, Wills, Durable Powers of Attorney, and an Advanced Health Care Directive. We learned that thorough consideration must be given to these documents at the onset—these specify who will be responsible for what, and includes naming an appropriate substitute should the primary candidate became unable to assume the responsibilities.

It is important to draw up the documents correctly to enable the designated person in charge to easily navigate the legalities that may ensue. Once the disease progresses, the patient will be unable to demonstrate competence, a new signature would be considered invalid (Venesa could not scrawl her initials, let alone sign her name), and some of the documentation can never be changed. It is essential to consult with a lawyer about this early on and understand the differences between documents and what specifically each confers!

Despite Venesa's having conferred her Durable Power of Attorney to me, it was insufficient to allow me to change some of her legal documentation later. In 2015 I tried to exercise my Durable Power of Attorney and Health Care Directive so as to add our son as a backup in the event that something were to happen to me and there would be no one to assume responsibility for Venesa. Legally, however, I learned that the only person who could make this change was Venesa herself and only if she could demonstrate to the lawyer and be certified that she knew what she was doing, why she was doing it, and that she was otherwise clear of mind. Of course by this time Venesa could not be certified and the documentation could not be legally changed.

Contingency Planning: The Alzheimer's Association reports that Alzheimer's dementia caregivers, put themselves at significant greater risk than do non-caregivers. This is a serious consideration that should be addressed as one plans and organizes for taking care of a loved one.

It is helpful to define the planning necessary for an immediate and smooth transition to caregiving once a person has been diagnosed so as to ensure that a patient is properly cared for, particularly in the event that the primary caregiver is hospitalized or passes away before the patient.

If living at home with a spouse or relative, where would the patient live? In my case, plans were established with a caregiving agency to leave Venesa in our house with full-time care for the rest of her life, with immediate implementation by the agency in the event of an emergency. Caregivers were instructed on providing all meals, feeding Venesa, and providing for all of her necessities, overseen by Debbie (the caregiver I eventually came to hire to help me as the disease progressed). Debbie would have been provided with a credit card—which would have been audited monthly by my son— with which to purchase the necessities such as food, medicine, clothes, diapers etc. All necessary transportation would have been provided by the caregivers using our specialized handicap vehicles, etc.

The finances had been set up to ensure the flow of money from retirement accounts and Social Security so that expenses could be paid by an ongoing automated system from my checking account. Additional funds were established for emergency expenses in a checking account (to be monitored by my son) to cover any major unexpected expenses in the event of my death or hospitalization. I purposely did *not* put this account into the trust to avoid the complexities in gaining access to money held in trust. Establishing a separate joint checking account would enable the second signer to easily access emergency funds. It is best to consult an estate planner early in the process and consider all possible contingencies as you set up your finances for retirement and future care. This will provide great peace of mind.

Housing: I promised Venesa that she would never be placed in a rest home and that she would always live in our house with me "until death do us part," as per our wedding vows. I committed to providing all care and support until things became particularly difficult, which they did in 2013 when I hired part-time support. But even with professional caregivers helping, I was able to keep this promise, and was generally with her at all times.

Logistics: The norm at the outset was to have Venesa accompany me on errands and other activities that took me away from home. As the disease progressed and toward the last two weeks, it became too difficult to bring her, so Venesa would stay with a caregiver while I provided for our necessities.

My Struggles as a Homemaker

Having been so focused on my career for many years, it was a slow realization that I, alone, would eventually be responsible for the complete care of the household and my spouse without the customary support Venesa had provided throughout our marriage. I was to assume all of Venesa's former responsibilities in addition to continuing my own. Fortunately, I had retired in 2007 while Venesa was still in Mild Cognitive Impairment (MCI) and I had a gradual increase in exposure to her responsibilities while she was still able to function. Upon retiring, I transitioned from being a program manager with responsibilities for launching satellites from both coasts to being a full-time caregiver—not easily done.

Cooking, shopping, planning balanced menus, laundry, house cleaning, sanitation, bathing, dressing, and maintaining Venesa's personal hygiene, coordinating her wardrobe, tending to hair and makeup, overseeing medications, and of course, tending to her (albeit declining) social life and mobility. One of the most difficult adjustments for me was the loss of her input in making life decisions, such as holiday plans, house decorations, financial planning, and such. And yet the hardest thing of all was the realization that I was losing my best friend, my lover, my co-parent, and my life companion.

Shopping and meal planning—This was a particular challenge as I did not want Venesa to lose weight that she might desperately need to sustain her if she were to be hospitalized. My strategy was to serve her favorite foods and, as time progressed and her appetite reduced, supplement her foods with Ensure Plus for additional nutrition and calories. Toward the end, she was drinking four to six bottles of Ensure Plus each day after eating her small meals.

I found that cooking is *not* rocket science—all you need is a good cookbook. Venesa's recipes and utensils were already available in the kitchen, although I did purchase a NutriBullet to make Venesa smoothies. I wrote the menus in advance, these served as guides for my grocery shopping, and I was careful to provide small servings that she could realistically consume and a variety of tastes and textures in each food group at each meal. I never knew what Venesa would accept at any particular meal, but as I learned as the disease progressed, she did not like her food pureed—instead I would cut it up for her as needed.

A typical day's menu would be:

Breakfast: Scrambled eggs with melted cheddar cheese; bacon, sausage, or ham; buttered toast with jelly or a Danish pastry; and orange juice as well as a bottle of Ensure Plus. At times the eggs would be replaced by pancakes or waffles with syrup, or I would prepare a well-fortified smoothie in the NutriBullet (with berries, frozen pineapple, protein powder, banana, strawberry Ensure Plus, pomegranate juice, and water).

Lunch: Homemade soup (such as beef bulgur, vegetable, or split pea), a buttered roll or toast, a serving of fruit, and a bottle of Ensure Plus. Sometimes the meal consisted of a sandwich (tuna salad or cold cuts with cheese), a serving of fruit and, of course, an Ensure Plus.

Dinner: A cut of meat (filet mignon, porterhouse, or New York strip steak), or baked chicken smothered in sautéed mushrooms and onions, ham, or barbecued salmon; then a baked potato, vegetables, fruit, Ensure Plus, and desert. Sometimes the meat or fish would be replaced by lasagna or some other pasta.

Sanitation and cleanliness—As time went on, there was a necessary increase in sanitation measures to ensure that Venesa remained healthy. For example I swept and steam-clean mopped her bathroom floor several times a week, vacuumed the carpet at least every other day, and steamed cleaned the carpet monthly. The kitchen floor was cleaned in a similar manner. A disinfectant cleaner with bleach was used liberally, painfully learning not to bleach things I did not want to turn white. Then there was the routine dusting and a variety of other household tasks.

Personal Care—Putting on Venesa's makeup, washing and combing her hair, hairdresser appointments, doctor appointments, and anticipating and maintaining supplies (such as diapers, special soaps, and hospital gowns that required internet ordering). As her disabilities increased, just giving Venesa shower became a monumental task. Getting her out of bed with the Hoyer lift and into a wheelchair, wheeling her into the bathroom, and the lift to get her from the wheelchair to the specialty shower chair, and rolling her into the shower; then lifting her back into the wheelchair and get her dressed for the day. Yes! the caregiving was challenging!

Personal interaction, respect, and intimacy—Venesa and I had always had a very close, intense relationship—both physically and emotionally—such that in losing her, I felt as if she has taken half my spirit and soul to heaven with her and left half of hers behind for me. We grew to be perfect soul mates and closest best friends, never even arguing. Instead we discussed differences of opinion, coming up with an acceptable solution for both of us. We had a total love and respect for one another, each willing to listen, try to understand the other's point of view, and compromise to reach an acceptable solution for both. Each of us tried to maximize the emotional support for the other's comfort and needs. We knew each other intimately, always discussed everything, and held nothing back, talking about values and bringing up the children, financial planning, where to live, sex, sports, friends, hopes, and frustrations. We held everything jointly—the deed to the house, titles for the cars, bank accounts, retirement accounts, and investments, providing for each other's future in the event of one of us having an early demise. Our emotions, possessions, and lives were completely intertwined. There was no reason to change this because of dementia. The difference was that, as the disease progressed, I would have to carry the load for both of us and take care to always respect the very caring foundations of our relationship and preserve Venesa's sense of dignity.

Once with very active libidos, we expressed our closeness, not only in the marital bed, but in our activities together, holding hands when we walked, massaging Venesa's scalp and back, accompanying each other on errands, social outings, and even out-of-town professional meetings. But in our 39th year of marriage, we began to experience some changes. Perhaps one of the first things I noticed was a total loss of Venesa's libido, followed shortly after by my own erectile dysfunction and low testosterone. It is unclear how much the emotional may have affected the physical or if it was somehow related to confronting the reality of Venesa's dementia. We addressed the erectile dysfunction with Viagra and the low testosterone with a prescription jelly that I rubbed on my shoulders and upper chest. Venesa never rejected our sexual encounters, but as time went on she did not seem comfortable with them. I discussed this with my primary care physician and he recommended we stop the activity because it might have been painful for Venesa. So we did and I stopped using Viagra.

My reaction to this new constraint was to do everything I could to express my love to Venesa so she would know the depth of my devotion to her. In bed, I would snuggle up to her, pull our bodies close together, give her big hugs and kisses, and tell her how much I loved her. But that was that! As time wore on the longing for our times together began to fade, but they never disappeared. The physical aspects took care of themselves. But as I began to feel the loneliness that progressively occupied the space that Venesa's personality had once filled, I found that distraction and activity were the most effective coping mechanisms.

Each day I networked with friends or combed through the local newspapers for announcements of events and planned outings to keep us active and provide stimulation for Venesa. While she was still able to participate in decision-making, I would consult with her as usual. But as the disease progressed, I had to rely on my knowing Venesa's likes and dislikes so well, and later on my ability to read her face, see in her eyes, her gestures, and physical emotions to know that she cared or tried to express intimacy, or that she was having a good time!

Outings and travel after diagnosis—Traveling, always a part of our lives, was to continue even after the diagnosis. There were major trips within the United States, one international trip, numerous day trips, and on days we were home without travel plans, we would take a walk in the local park, the neighborhood, or golf course for about one hour and a half. We also actually "played" golf or tennis (according to her changing abilities), and of course there were our shopping trips and errands. During inclement weather, we would just walk in the big box stores or at the mall.

Day trips were always stimulating. We often went to visit one of the local zoos, to see the ocean and the large population of elephant seals, to see the butterflies swarming, lunch at a favorite seaside restaurant, the local strawberry or avocado festivals, the Elks rodeo, a Renaissance fair, to feed the animals on display at the Avila Barn country market, to vintage car shows, the Mexican Fiesta in nearby Santa Barbara, among other events in the vicinity.

Coping with Loneliness and Depression

At the outset, I decided that giving in to loneliness and depression was not an option for me. As Venesa's agent in her Advanced Healthcare Directive, she had directed me to "allow me [Venesa] to die as gently as possible" even if in doing so it would hasten her death.

To honor this direction, I did everything possible to keep her comfortable, pain free, and happy throughout the entire progression of the disease. And, honoring this directive required that I maintain a "a stiff upper lip" and somehow always appear to be positive and upbeat, particularly because Venesa was so aware of her surroundings up to the end. Although she could not always express herself, her demeanor told me she understood. I also recognized that, although depression was a natural reaction to our predicament, indulging myself in lamentation would ultimately be counterproductive to both of us. Intent on counteracting a negative reaction I sought relief in prayer, thanking God for his divine intervention and in counting my many blessings:

1. For having had 43 years of a wonderful marriage to a true friend, lover, and soulmate who was a true asset to society as a professor, mentor, and philanthropist.
2. For having had the resources that provided for fulfillment during those 43 years.
3. For Venesa's having overcome breast cancer when our sons were 2 and 7. Venesa had worried so much that someone else might have to raise our sons. We were blessed that the surgery was successful.
4. For God having allowed me to overcome a burst appendix and massive gangrene in my chest cavity at age 21. I recognized that had this occurred only a couple of years

earlier, before penicillin was developed, it would have been fatal.
5. For having shared the opportunity with Venesa to watch and guide our two wonderful sons from birth to become productive members of society. Although both had married by the time she was in the moderate middle stage of dementia, she had met and known both wives, as well as the joy of having two grandchildren.
6. And foremost, for God's having given me the fortitude and the resources to be able to care for Venesa and provide the best for her, to implement creative solutions to meet her needs, and to maintain her mobility, emotions, and general quality of life.

And yet, with all the divine intervention and my recognition of these blessings, I can't deny that there was a deep, sad, loneliness and depression encroaching upon me as the disease progressed and Venesa became more remote. I had to constantly remind myself of my blessings to keep on track and stay as upbeat as possible—it was not easy—and it was not sufficient!

I found that staying active, distracted, and having a sense of purpose augmented my religious foundation and helped to keep loneliness and depression at bay. Having Debbie, our seasoned caregiver, also helped tremendously during the last year and a half. Clearly, she impacted our lives. Her partnering with me in caregiving, her discussions, and her suggestions helped me stay upbeat and positive; her friendship through caregiving was exceptional.

Since I had committed to regular outings, travel, and making sure Venesa was stimulated and exercised, I enthusiastically threw myself into planning our days. Having scanned the newspaper for activities and events, virtually every morning before Venesa woke up I would discuss the day's activities with

Debbie. The planning itself seemed to take my mind away from the disease for a while, giving me a sense of purpose for the day and anticipation of the future adventures. Further, the challenges entailed in the logistics of taking care of Venesa's personal needs provided distraction and kept me active and away from my thoughts. Fundamentally, I just stayed busy.

The outings were always entertaining—errands, lunches out, exercise sessions, excursions, and trips. Trying to stay sane, I began to attend an Alzheimer's Association support group for caregivers. However, because Venesa and I seemed to be further along in our journey through the disease, it seemed I did most of the talking, supporting others through sharing my experiences, while not feeling that I was particularly unburdened or supported. In the evenings, I relaxed with a cocktail (mindful to stay alert so as not to put Venesa at risk if she were to need help); I had dinner and watched TV news after Venesa went to bed. And while I was alone in those quiet moments, I never allowed myself to feel the depth of the obvious loneliness—remembering always that I was blessed.

Coping with the Progression of LBD Dementia

Exercise

Exercise has been shown to be extremely important to maintaining a high quality of life for all people, and particularly for the dementia patient.

Through exercise, core muscles are developed to maintain body posture and strength, and muscular toning , allows for pain-free body movement that is necessary for all activities— walking, lifting, sports such as golf and tennis, exercise programs such as tai chi or yoga, dancing—providing general freedom both in and outdoors to participate in whatever activities are enjoyable to the patient. Cognitive activity is stimulated 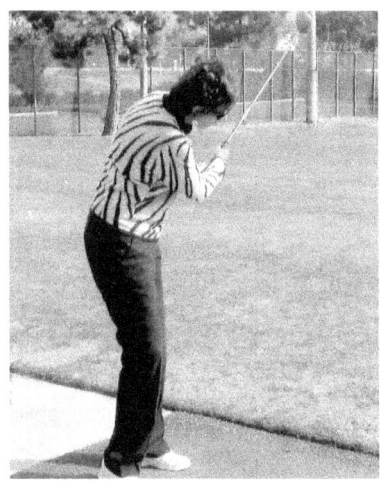 through exercise, requiring mental focus, strategy development, rapid creative thinking. For example, should you aim a golf shot over the trees or take a more conservative approach around the trees? What club do you use to achieve your objective? Should a tennis shot be a drop shot? Should it be approached with forehand with spin on the ball? Should it be returned with a backhand?

Cardiovascular health is also developed and maintained through exercise, particularly through brisk walking, jogging, and running (outdoors, on a treadmill, or on an elliptical machine) or bicycle riding or rowing. Taking the importance of exercise into consideration, the caregiver for a person with LBD must strive to maintain the patient's quality of life as long as the disease will permit. Thus, it is essential to incorporate exercise into the patient's routine for as long as the patient's condition will permit, perhaps modifying the activity to meet the patient's declining abilities. I believe this can extend the patient's life.

I made an effort to keep Venesa flexible and increase her hand-to-eye coordination and balance by teaching her to play golf and continuing the tennis she had always played. Venesa had played golf only two or three times in her life, but beginning in 2012, she took a series of lessons from a professional golfer at the local country club. With Venesa's athletic background, she took to the game with gusto. The lessons initially took place at the driving range and eventually included golfing on the course. Since she could not drive the ball much more than 60 to 80 yards, we started by teeing off halfway down the fairway and playing the remainder of the hole, including chipping and putting. She learned what club was to be used where and seemed to truly enjoy the lessons. We continued with this activity until 2013, when the golf pro left the club. Before playing golf and in parallel with her golf lessons, Venesa played tennis.

Venesa was an ex-club champion and had been a well-respected player. We played tennis well into 2015 even after she was wheelchair bound. Wheeling Venesa onto the court, I would stand her up at the back of the court and loosely hold onto the back of her gait belt for security, prepared to gently lower her to the ground if she were to lose her balance. A caregiver would stand on the other side of the net and feed her 100 to 120 balls. She would step into the ball (forehand and backhand) and hit 80 to 90 percent of the balls back over the net. Her muscle memory was incredible, she remained significantly flexible, she lost her balance only once, and she benefited from the activity and being outdoors.

While she didn't swim often, she did have occasion to enjoy an outdoor swimming pool in 2015 (while in Houston). She would swim under water (while I held her for safety), relishing the experience.

Mobility

Although Venesa's mobility had already been somewhat impaired before LBD had been diagnosed, it became increasingly difficult as the disease progressed. Venesa's mobility problems had started with her arthroscopic knee surgery in 1989, a partial knee replacement in 2010, and total knee replacement of both knees in 2011. Her inability to easily walk from her office to class in another building and stand lecturing for an hour or more had actually prompted her retirement from California Polytechnic University in 2010. After recovering from her surgeries, she was able to walk reasonably well for short activities in the house, at the park, and around the neighborhood. Her walking was impacted by the dementia itself in early 2013, when she was in mid-stage LBD. Although she continued to walk, it was with assistance from a caregiver and for short distances only. Because of her cognitive impairment, she was never able to master the use of a cane or a walker of any kind. She perceived of walking aids as stable support structures and would depend on them for stability, unable to grasp the concept that they were to be used for support during movement. We would walk with her in the house, but by 2014 she transitioned into a wheelchair when we went for our walks outside.

Venesa's ability to walk became further impacted in 2015 when she began to freeze and seemingly want to walk on tiptoes only. With that, we transitioned her to a wheelchair inside the house. By November of that year her mobility was strictly limited to the wheelchair and we had to utilize the Hoyer lift for all transitions between the wheelchair, bed, shower, and lavatory.

As her walking declined, it became much more difficult for me to get Venesa in and out of the car. So, by the latter portion of her mid-stage (2013) we replaced the passenger seat of our van with a "valet" disability car seat. This seat provided a support mechanism to ease a person into or out of the car.

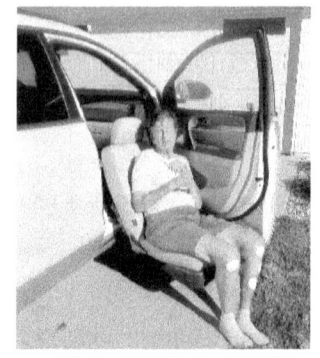

Within about a year and a half, when she approached mid-late stage LBD, even this became too difficult and, in early 2015, I purchased a wheelchair van such that she could be wheeled into the car without the need to stand up or change seats. One side of the van would lower down and provide a ramp with which to wheel her in and out of the car. The car was equipped to automatically lock her wheelchair into the passenger side, enabling us to continue our outings.

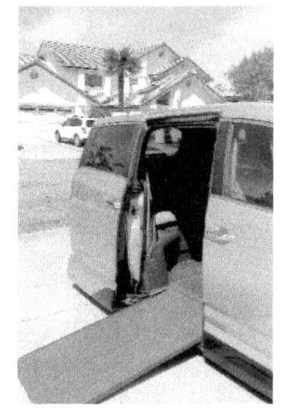

Medications

Beyond the obvious responsibility of purchasing and dispensing her medications, it was important to make sure Venesa took her routine medications on schedule. From the early diagnosis of the disease and throughout its progression, our doctors were adamant about not using any type or quantity of medication that could not be demonstrated to be absolutely necessary and beneficial to Venesa. Because all medications can have side effects, the premise for prescribing a medication was to find a balance between its potential effectiveness in resolving a problem and the presence/absence of collateral effects. The intent was to only use medications that were absolutely necessary at a dose that had favorable results and that didn't require another medication to counteract an unintended side effect.

This approach was implemented throughout the progression of the disease, and when Venesa passed she was taking only four prescription and three over-the-counter medications. There were weeks, however, when short-term medications were required and I had to learn how to administrate them. Prior to and after surgeries, I gave her a daily shot of Lovenox in her lower abdomen as a bridge for Coumadin. For several weeks I gave her very strong intravenous antibiotics to fight infection—antibiotics so strong that its strength was adjusted each week on the basis of a current blood test by the Infusion Services Lab. Then there were treatments for the all-too-frequent UTIs, bouts with pneumonia and, of course, pain management. I certainly had never expected that I would learn to provide this level of medical attention!

Incontinence

By the latter part of Venesa's moderate middle stage of LBD, she began to experience urinary incontinence; bowel incontinence followed during her severe late stage. In general, the pull-up panty diapers worked well until Venesa's mobility became such that she was not able to stand up to put them on; the wrap-around diapers were then put into play. She had such volume that we had to use the top-of-the-line most absorbent diapers we could find, which were not available locally but could be ordered online. Even at that, she overflowed the diapers several times while we were in Houston.

Dealing with Venesa's incontinence was a very different experience for me, but as with all other aspects of my caregiving, I learned to cope with it well. Naturally, with all our outings we needed to use public restrooms in restaurants, airports, fair grounds, and many other public places. We used family restrooms when they were available. Normally these contained one commode, no urinal, and plenty of room for a wheelchair. These were infrequently available and usually found only in new or recently restored public facilities such as airports and shopping centers. If a family restroom was not available, we had the choice of using the men's room, which normally had a handicap commode in a stall. But because we would have to walk past men using a stand-up urinal with minimal privacy, we never used these. The enclosed stalls in the women's room, on the other hand, generally provided a handicapped stall, so the women's room was much preferred. Happily, in all of the times we used the women's rooms in public places, I never encountered a woman that was upset by my presence. Quite the opposite, women usually offered to help in any way they could.

One of the biggest challenges with Venesa's incontinence was in the multiple times she needed to be tested for a urinary tract infection. The urine in the diaper could not be used because it was considered contaminated and, because of her incontinence, she could not provide a urine sample for testing. She had to have a catheter inserted to draw the sample.

Nothing is Impossible—
Journeying with Dementia

Traveling with a person who has dementia typically becomes more difficult because the progression of the disease is accompanied by decreased function and greater disorientation and anxiety. Nonetheless, Venesa and I had determined to continue activities that had always been meaningful to us. Traveling was at the top of our list, but of course, adjustments had to be made. 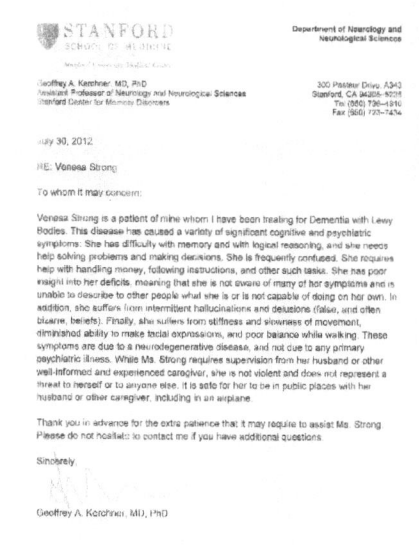 Airline travel was more convoluted and required significantly more planning and preparation. When we asked Dr. Kerchner about the feasibility of travel, he encouraged us by saying "Go for it," but suggested I carry a letter with his explanation of Venesa's illness. He was concerned about Venesa's possible confusion in clearing the TSA check or customs check. Dr. Kerchner provided me with a letter identifying Venesa as his patient and describing the possible unusual behaviors she might exhibit, while stating that it was safe for her to travel with me, and requesting that the reader have extra patience to assist me. The letter was formal and written on Stanford School of Medicine letterhead.

For travel by air, we checked our own wheelchair through as baggage and took advantage of the airlines' wheelchair service to compensate for Venesa's slow pace, difficulty walking, and inability to stand in the long check-in, TSA, and customs lines.

This service prioritizes disabled passengers, allowing them to move through the processes more quickly. Further, we used the service to transport her between gates for connecting flights, which often took us through employee-only areas and significantly shortened the distance between gates.

On the plane, air travel required that we use First Class bulkhead seating, as this is the roomiest seating on the aircraft and, in reality, it would have been nearly impossible to get her in and out of any other seating. For the flight itself, Venesa was transferred to a disability aisle wheelchair to be used inside the plane. The airline sometimes provided up to four support personnel to transfer her from the aisle wheelchair to her seat or back to a wheelchair that the airlines provided at the arrival gate.

Once at our final destination, the airline wheelchair service would meet us at the plane and take us to baggage claim where we would pick up the wheelchair we had checked through baggage, Venesa would then be transferred to that and we left for ground transportation to our final destination.

In terms of ground transportation, we learned that Venesa was not able to use the taxi system because the cars have thick security barriers between the front and rear seats, reducing the foot room in the back. Venesa literally could not get into the back seat in any way, not even sitting sideways. However, the ground transportation ordered in advance for a handicapped person enabled her to ride comfortably.

Our travels between July 2011 (with moderate stage dementia) and June 2015 (with late stage dementia) were motivated by family events, professional and educational opportunities, and a sense of adventure. Some of the trips were relatively uneventful, others were more challenging.

Traveling with Moderate Stage Dementia
July 2011; Philadelphia, Chicago, and Cedarburg; Family Travel

Our youngest son had just purchased a home in Philadelphia (PA), and Venesa had wanted to see it. Believing that, "there is no time like the present," with the blessing of Dr. Kerchner, we flew from our home in Santa Maria to see the new house, visit our son and his future wife, and spend the weekend sightseeing in historic downtown Philadelphia.

   To get an overview of what there was to see and determine what our priorities would be, we sat on the open upper level of a double-decker tour bus to maximize our view, which unfortunately also provided maximum sun exposure. After alighting the bus downtown, I left Venesa seated on a comfortable window seat in an air-conditioned building and went to the other side of the room to pick up tickets for the buildings and exhibits we wanted to see. Alarmed, Venesa called out to tell me she did not feel right. As I helped her to the water cooler, she passed out, and I gently let her slip down to the floor. The security guard helped me get her up and comfortable, and assisted me in calling a cab to take her to the hospital. Venesa was admitted to the hospital with severe dehydration and she was kept for observation and testing. While there was no ostensible problem diagnosed, I think the temperature difference from the very hot outside to the cold air conditioning may have caused Venesa to faint. With that, I learned the importance of flexibility in traveling—one must be prepared to change plans as necessity dictates.

   Medical scientists are increasingly recognizing early changes often observed in LBD within the autonomic nervous system. These features, albeit subtle in some cases, often become apparent well before other clinical manifestations are present. Perhaps the most substantial and serious change revolves around loss of the distribution of nerves (innervation) within the sympathetic portion of the autonomic nervous system that regulates heart rate and blood pressure. Typically, individuals with this LBD feature note lightheadedness when standing suddenly and may actually faint (syncope); the lowering of blood pressure when ascending against gravity is known as orthostatic hypotension. When not changing position, blood pressure may be normal or high; the impairment is in the *regulation* of dynamic changes.

Venesa was released from the hospital the next day and the incident did not deter us from enjoying the balance of our time with our son or prevent us from visiting other relatives in Chicago (IL), and Cedarburg (WI). My sister's oldest daughter, Ellen, showed us the sights in Chicago and then we visited with my sister and the rest of her family in Cedarburg and the wilderness of the family cabin on Chute Pond in upstate Wisconsin. Happily, Venesa was fully active, riding a

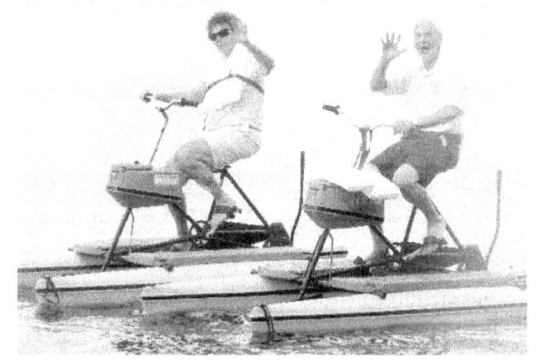

single-passenger bicycle boat, swimming, and kayaking—enjoying the surroundings and our time with family.

August 2011; Venesa's Birthday, Wild Animal Park (CA); Family Travel

Venesa's 70th birthday was August 7. Kristin, our daughter-in-law, had a superb idea. Several times Venesa had made reservations and paid for a private-jet African safari to see the animals in Africa in their natural surroundings. Each time the trip had to be cancelled—the financial crisis of 2008, the twin tower catastrophe on 9/11, among other complications. By 2011 her deteriorating health made it unlikely that she would ever be able to fulfill this desire. So Kristin said, "If Venesa cannot go to Africa on safari why not bring Africa to her?" and she proceeded to organize a surprise birthday party for Venesa at the San Diego Wild Animal Park. This park lets the animals wander through acres of a simulated natural habitat, contained only by natural boundaries they will not cross.

Elaborate plans were made to rent flatbed trucks to transport our guests; provide guides to drive, oversee, and explain the tour through the park, as well as provide food for us to hand-feed the animals and see them up close; learn about and pet some rare small animals; enjoy a birthday dinner catered by the park in one of their grass huts; and, of course to surprise Venesa.

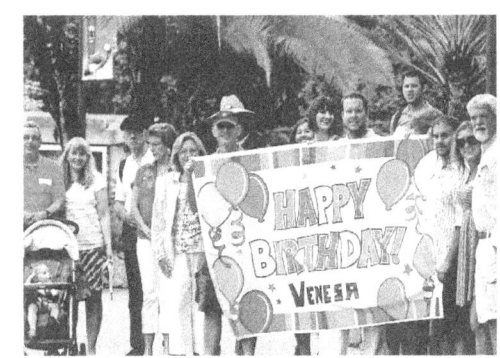

The plan went flawlessly and Venesa was nicely surprised to see many of her friends holding a huge sign "Happy Birthday Venesa" as we entered the park. Venesa had a fabulous day feeding some of the animals, seeing them in their natural habitats, feasting in the grass hut, and playing games. No unusual incidents, happy times, great memories!

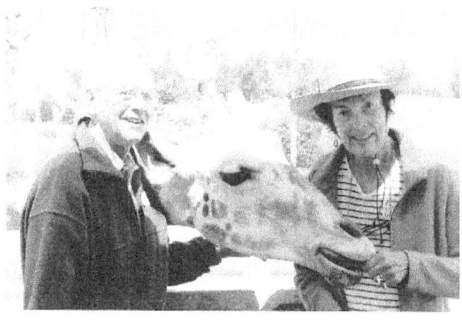

November 2011; Irvine (CA); Educational Travel
Venesa had just been diagnosed with LBD six months earlier and, of course, we knew very little about the disease. We found a series of educational sessions held by the University of Irvine at their facility just five hours from our home. I decided we would attend the series. I clearly benefitted greatly from these sessions, learning about the cause, the state of current research and the future of cure, and what to expect with the progression of the disease. I passed this information to my children. As an aside, I strongly recommend that anybody whose life is touched by dementia take advantage of the many educational opportunities offered by the Alzheimer's Association, generally at no cost.

December 2011; San Francisco (CA); Personal Travel
Venesa managed to negotiate social spaces well on her own as late as 2011, when we attended a formal birthday party at the Top of the Mark in San Francisco for Phyllis, one of her high school friends. Venesa had been very close to Phyllis and was seated with her at the front table, while I was seated elsewhere. I did not see any reason to inform anyone at the party that Venesa had been diagnosed with LBD because it did not seem to me to be that obvious. However, after the party Phyllis commented to me that there was nothing behind her eyes when they talked, that Venesa was cognitively absent. Phyllis was clearly shocked. Phyllis had anticipated in-depth conversation to "catch up" on things after a long separation—which could not happen because of Venesa's disease. In retrospect it would probably have been better if I had told Phyllis before the party and briefly explained what Venesa's situation was. If I had, perhaps Phyllis may have made other seating arrangements for the dinner. I do not know if Venesa caused any disruption during the dinner.

2011–2015; San Diego, Houston, Philadelphia, Atlanta San Jose, and Riverside; Travel for Professional Meetings
Throughout Venesa's professional life, she had been active in the Academy of Nutrition and Dietetics and the California Academy of Nutrition and Dietetics, serving as head of media relations, newsletter editor, head of the Consulting Dietitians subgroup, among other positions, before she became afflicted with LBD. After I retired I accompanied her to both organizations' meetings, where she was a full participant in each session. She continued to attend even after diagnosis, although her ability to understand the research and communicate with people gradually deteriorated over time. Each meeting focused on four full days of professional lectures, meetings with friends and colleagues from all over the country and state, from 7 a.m. to 6 p.m., hearing updates on the most current research. She had attended these faithfully for years for professional development, and we thought that her familiarity with the content and the professional community would be helpful in keeping her mind active and stimulated. She derived much pleasure from updating her contacts with old friends and associates, and the meetings did help her cognitively. In 2014 both the California Chapter and the National Organization recognized her for 50 years of service as a Registered Dietitian.

September 2012; The Beautiful Blue Danube—A River Trip from Hungary to Nuremberg to the Czech Republic; Adventure Travel
Perhaps our biggest trip—and our most challenging—was the river cruise we took down the Blue Danube. Although by this time Venesa was unable to express her desire for the trip, knowing her love for travel and adventure, I made the reservations. I had long since learned to read her emotions and facial expressions by the time I proposed this trip. The initial trip

(from Santa Maria to Budapest) required going through customs, and a layover at Heathrow Airport (London) for several hours, stretching the trip to 34 hours.

    This trip was taken approximately 18 months after she was diagnosed, in the middle stage of LBD. Although she could still walk with difficulty she required substantial help; cognitively, she could follow directions, but she could not carry on a reasonable conversation. Reasoning by this time was virtually nonexistent.

    During the flight Venesa became agitated for the first time (possibly due to disorientation). Undoubtedly this was triggered by the television monitors on the plane that were never turned off and prevented her from sleeping. She had complained about this several times. When we arrived in Budapest we went to the hotel, checked in, and were scheduled to sleep for about four hours before touring the city. However, Venesa was only able to sleep for a couple of hours. We got up and dressed to go to a lavish buffet breakfast, but Venesa would have no part of it. Undoubtedly disoriented, she again became agitated. All she would do was pace the hotel hallways—she refused to return to the room, partake of the buffet, let me partake of the buffet, or even sit down to have a cup of coffee. I had no medication to help alleviate this situation and all I could do was comfort her and generally accommodate her desires with patience. Finally, after 4.5 hours of walking, I was able to coax Venesa back to our room and she managed to sleep. Yes, we missed the Budapest tour.

    When she finally got up she was feeling so poorly that I had the hotel call in a doctor (who arrived on a bicycle with all his medical equipment in a backpack). With his limited diagnostic capabilities on site, he suggested transport to a hospital where she could better be tested and diagnosed. An ambulance was called to take her to a modern hospital, where a neurologist was called to consult despite the midnight hour. Physically, Venesa was deemed well enough to take the cruise the next day. Although we never did get to tour Budapest, there were eight other cities and the countryside along the river to see.

We stopped at Vienna, Durnstein, Melk, Linz, Passau, Regensburg, and Nuremberg on the river tour and we then took a motor coach to Prague. While staying in Prague, Venesa surprised me by going down to the front desk and telling the desk clerk that she was being held hostage in her room. Fortunately, I was right behind her with a copy of the letter from Dr. Kerchner. After reading it, the desk clerk nodded and handed it back to me. Thanks to Dr. Kerchner's foresight, a very difficult situation had been averted. I was deeply relieved.

The travel agency was particularly accommodating in each city, providing bus transportation for passengers who were unable to participate in the walking tours at each city. One city did not have busses so we were driven around in a children's train that was big enough to seat adults. We flew home from Prague without incident until the final leg of the trip from San Francisco to Santa Barbara. When we were waiting to board the aircraft Venesa announced that she was not going to board the plane—a comment that the pilot and head stewardess (also waiting for the plane) overheard. They had both experienced Alzheimer's with their parents, recognized my dilemma, and did a wonderful job convincing Venesa to board the plane albeit in an unconventional way—immediately after the arriving passengers alighted the plane even before the crew started to prepare the plane for the next flight. Venesa was comfortably settled into her seat well before the rest of the passengers boarded the plane.

Traveling with Late Stage Dementia
August 2013, Philadelphia; January 2015, Cedarburg; Family Travel

In 2013 we again traveled to Philadelphia to celebrate the marriage of our youngest son. The wedding was at a restaurant on a large boat that was docked on the river in central Philadelphia. Happily, the flight, accommodations, the visit, and the festivities were uneventful.

After my sister's death in January 2015, Venesa and I went to Cedarburg for the memorial services. Venesa was able to talk, given she had a few moments to collect her thoughts. She understood we were at my sister's funeral and recognized all family participants. Anne, one of my sister's daughters asked Venesa if she recognized her and, with her dry sense of humor, Venesa said "Why yeah" (like it was a no brainer). The family went out of its way to keep her included in the conversation and comfortable.

Due to inclement weather and Venesa's advancing LBD, traveling was a real challenge. By this point, Venesa was already dependent on the wheelchair, but with ice and snow even the wheelchair was difficult to maneuver. The return trip home turned out to be a particular challenge. Snow and ice had closed the Milwaukee airport and roads to Chicago were barely passable. My sister's daughter-in-law, Shannon, braved the storm to drive us to the Chicago O'Hare Airport, which fortunately remained open just long enough for us to catch our flight home.

Venesa had a very high cognitive ability during this entire trip. Airline travel to and from Chicago, automobile transportation in Illinois and Wisconsin went without a hitch as far as Venesa's abilities and cooperation. There was no indication of disorientation or concern on Venesa's part. Even the hotel, with the frigid temperatures, the snow and ice outside did not throw Venesa off. Venesa slept well, seemed completely comfortable, and was very cooperative.

June, 2015; Our Final Trip: Houston; Travel for Friends
On our final trip, a trip to Houston (Texas) to visit Venesa's closest friends, I recognized for the first time that Venesa was beginning to struggle with the process of traveling. We had flown to Houston for Venesa to visit friends who dated back to their days of shared internship training and early employment, and they became roommates.

Travel itself was difficult—particularly getting in and out of cars. Venesa wasn't able to sit upright in her wheelchair, leaning heavily to one side or the other. She was unable to talk. She was incontinent and seemed to overflow even her specialty diapers, leaving a pool on the floor when we transferred her into her wheelchair, and again when she exited the limousine—despite having been completely changed in between.

Venesa did seem to recognize her friends, although she did not call them by name and had little interaction with them. The visit generally went well, particularly the inclusiveness of swimming in the local Olympic-size pool, which was especially adapted for adults with disabilities. The pool was only five-feet deep and had a wide concrete entrance ramp with a gentle slope to provide easy access. I held on to Venesa the entire time we were in the pool. Although Venesa had been quite the swimmer throughout her life and with muscle memory she tried to paddle, but I was not comfortable allowing her to swim freely. She really enjoyed the experience—dunking under water and just playing in the pool. A great time was had by all.

All in all, I recognized that I was probably pushing the travel experience too hard and, once home, this should probably be the final major trip.

Maintaining Skills in the Face of Decline

Throughout the entire progression of the disease, it seemed as though we were constantly in and out of outpatient physical therapy trying to keep Venesa as flexible and independent as possible, and happy. However, 2013 was particularly challenging. During this year, we not only took her to aggressive physical therapy but also added a Ph.D. speech language pathologist to increase her ability to "find" the right words, help her enunciation, and improve her associated cognitive function. Exercises to help her recognize friends and family, as well as recognize common household items were included. Helping her to eat and swallow were continually evaluated due to a concern for potential aspiration.

By the third quarter of 2013, Venesa was not responding to the therapies as well as we thought she should and we were at the Medicare physical therapy funding limits for that particular year. Upon the recommendation of her physical therapist, Venesa's primary care physician referred her to a local rehabilitation hospital. The hospital's evaluation of Venesa's needs suggest she be admitted for a 10-day "tune up."

Venesa's stay was planned, directed, and monitored by the medical director, who specialized in physical medicine, rehabilitation, rehabilitation pain medicine, and brain injury. This was an aggressive inpatient hospital program that included three lengthy therapy sessions each day (physical therapy, speech therapy, and an occupational therapy session).

The physical therapy was individualized for each patient to achieve improvement and maximize effectivity. The exercises were very appropriate and creative, each focusing on a particular need within the physical therapy realm.

The speech therapy program was also aggressive and included methods to help find the right word, improve diction, recognize familiar individuals as well as food textures, and to avoid aspiration pneumonia.

The occupational therapy program focused on activities of daily life, including skills to participate in dressing, bathing, and eating. The classes stressed skills to use implements such as knives, forks, and spoons with special handles to aid in grasping them. Specialized implements were also available to help put on socks. These skills were also reinforced during physical therapy sessions.

Above and beyond the planned activities, Dr. Harbaugh was brought in for a neurological evaluation of Venesa; his findings and recommendations for supporting Venesa's needs were extremely helpful. In between her classes Venesa and I would walk around the facility (with the permission of the medical director) to gain additional strength.

The hospital provided gourmet meals from an outside vendor with a multiple-choice menu for the patients. While I was able to join Venesa at mealtime with my own takeout meal from the hospital cafeteria, the rooms were shared rooms and I was unable to stay with her overnight. However, the hospital did have cottages to accommodate the patient's visiting relatives on an as-available basis, asking for a donation of "what you feel is right." These were very clean, neat, and functional, located very close to the hospital.

Since Venesa had slept with me in a king-size bed for so many years, I was concerned about how she might react if she were to wake up in the middle of the night and not find me there. The cottages were close enough that I could be there within a couple of minutes if needed, which gave me comfort. However, this was not an issue; the hospital worked hard to maximize patient comfort and provide a positive hospital experience, and Venesa was indeed comfortable and appreciative.

Choosing Caregiver Support

Until 2013 I had successfully managed to be with Venesa literally 24 hours each day 7 days a week. But I began to recognize that I needed help. I went to the local Area Council for the Aging to get a list of potential caregiving agencies. Initially I generated a list of my requirements and sent it out for "bid." This, however, resulted in responses from only two agencies. I selected one and tried it part time, but it really did not work. The three or four different caregivers from that agency simply did not relate well with Venesa. The owner of the agency constrained the services that the caregivers were permitted to provide due to a concern over their sustaining personal injury from straining. Further, we differed in perspectives over the freedom of movement that Venesa was allowed to have, with the agency trying to limit it against my instructions to maximize it. By 2014, I had replaced the first agency with a new one.

The second agency was also problematic. After trying three or four of their caregivers, I found that none could relate well to Venesa or help her mobility. Venesa was 6 feet tall and of relatively large frame—not fat—just a large beautiful lady. The agency philosophy was apparently to send "revolving caregivers" rather than the same caregiver for each visit. This seemed to confuse Venesa; she could not bond with the rotating caregivers and, from the very lack of familiarity, the caregiver was not able to recognize Venesa's subtle changes that might require immediate medical attention.

Having experienced difficulties with hiring multiple caregivers from each of the first two caregiving agencies, the depth of Venesa's needs and desires began to crystalize in my mind. If something were to happen to me, I needed to have an agency that was capable of providing complete care and a person to oversee that Venesa's needs were well met. Thus, my new quest was to contract a single caregiver that would be able to assume all of my responsibilities, stepping into the lead if I were to be unable to continue caregiving. With that firmly in mind, I required that the next agency provide a single caregiver for up to 40 hours a week, rejecting the idea of revolving caregivers. I was willing to consider a second caregiver if our caregiving needs exceeded 40 hours. My rationale for this was as follows:

- Deep trust and confidence could be established, such that Venesa would feel comfortable (safety concerns, toileting, dressing, etc.)
- The caregiver's personality and temperament could be aligned to Venesa's
- The caregiver would have greater familiarity with the progression of the disease in Venesa, and would better recognize subtleties that might indicate a change in treatment (recognize UTIs or illnesses, eating disorders, expressions of emotions or pain)

I then engaged a third agency in November 2014. Although this agency had told me that its normal policy was to send revolving caregivers, it had just hired a caregiver with 30 years' experience (and some experience with dementia with LBD—a very difficult find) who was adamant about working with a single client only. The owner of the agency recognized how ideal a pairing it would make, and indeed, the match was a fabulous success. Venesa and Debbie bonded well with each other.

By the fourth quarter of 2015, however, it was apparent that I needed even more help. By then Venesa's mobility was entirely dependent on using the Hoyer Lift and I had gotten two compression fractures on my spine from trying to lift Venesa. She had done exactly what I had requested but, unfortunately, I had given her incorrect instructions.

With this, Debbie and I began the hunt for a second caregiver to work as a backup and to take over two days per week, providing me with support the entire week. After interviewing (and trying out) multiple caregivers, we were fortunate to find another perfect fit for Venesa's personality and her particular needs, Natalie. Although Natalie had no caregiving experience, she had run a childcare facility and was extremely patient; she was a fast learner and was solidly grounded with common sense. Debbie trained Natalie very quickly.

I found that professional caregivers' observations could be more astute than my own. Being around Venesa so constantly, changes could go unperceived by me. However, with the caregivers being part-time only, they could recognize changes more readily; for example, urinary tract infections could be detected earlier and treated more quickly. We were an effective and well-balanced team that Venesa responded to positively and loved.

Debbie and Natalie remained with us until Venesa passed. They were gratefully appreciated.

Ongoing Adaptations in the Face of Ongoing Decline

Adapting the Environment

The furniture, window coverings, and decor in our home had been updated the last half of 2013, accommodating some of Venesa's needs. We had purchased a new zero-gravity leather recliner for Venesa at that time. While it was very comfortable for her, the back did not have wings so she would lean over to her right or left and end up supported by the relatively low arms of the chair in what looked like a particularly uncomfortable position. 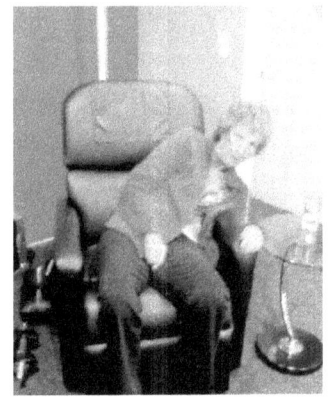 When we tried to get her to sit up straight she would just lean over more. She had lost the ability to sit upright! So in March 2014 we had a padded eight-inch wing added to each side of the chair by a custom upholsterer, to support her properly. The addition was perfect; the chair looked like it came that way from the factory and it provided the necessary support for Venesa to sit upright comfortably.

Using Debbie's very strong caregiving background, I followed her recommendations on adapting the environment to enable Venesa to remain mobile and active. Over time, we added:

- A ramp to transport Venesa in and out of the garage. This was an immediate need; Venesa was still walking with difficulty but we knew a wheelchair was in her future.
- An electric Hoyer lift and proper slings. Initially the lift was considered to be an emergency backup to move Venesa, but we knew that it would be put to good use as

the disease progressed. The electric lift gives the caregiver much better control than the pump-type Hoyer lift, as the caregiver can actively help the patient and simultaneously operate the lift.
- A medical air mattress was mandatory to prevent decubitus ulcers. To be effective, the mattress must be sized to the patient and have alternating pressure low-air loss. The alternating pressure would gently increase the pressure on Venesa's back from her right side to her left side then back again every 15 minutes throughout the night or whenever it was in use. The low-air loss maintains a cool temperature for the patient, and is a vast improvement over the standard use of pillows to shift from side to side, as was done each time Venesa was in the hospital. Venesa would always return home with one or more decubitus ulcers after several days in the hospital; this mattress would resolve them within two days!
- A custom wheelchair was required for Venesa's comfort because she was a larger than average person. Further, she used a ROHO air-inflatable cushion on the seat of her wheelchair for comfort and to minimize decubitus ulcers.
- A sliding shower chair provided safety, comfort, and ease of showering. Debbie and I both believed that Venesa deserved a real shower with the scalp massage she loved while her hair was being washed, as well as all of the other comforts of the shower process. A sponge bath in bed was unacceptable to us and we provided showers to the end.
- As Venesa's mobility deteriorated, we obtained a hospital bed through Medicare to make her care easier, safer, and more comfortable.

Throughout our marriage Venesa and I had always slept together. With the arrival of the hospital bed I replaced our king-sized bed with the hospital bed, placing a twin bed for me close to it. A couple of days after this new sleeping arrangement was done, Venesa commented several times to Debbie (but never to me), "I have been a bad girl." When Debbie told me about this, we tried to figure out what might be wrong. Debbie suggested pushing the two beds together, leveling the height of the hospital bed to the twin bed. While we made up each bed separately with mattress pads and contoured sheets for comfort and functionality, we used a king-sized top sheet and the familiar blankets and comforter Venesa and I had used for years. The problem was solved with these more familiar surroundings—Venesa seemed much happier and never mentioned the "bad girl" statement again.

This is a sterling example of the benefits of having an experienced caregiver that can think outside the box. I never would have imagined the source of the problem nor would I have resolved the dilemma quite so practically.

We also purchased clothing (hospital gowns with open backs), bibs to use during meals and decorative bibs to catch drooling, and highly absorbent stretch briefs, among other things. Special deep-cleaning aids were purchased to clean up after accidents and to maintain a sterile environment (carpet shampooer, steam cleaner for the marble and tile floors, special sanitary wood floor cleaners disinfectant window cleaners, and counter cleaners).

We knew Venesa would never be bed bound for any significant amount of time and that she would live at home in a sanitary environment.

We were well prepared!

Adapting to a Variety of Medical Needs
The progression of LBD demanded that we accommodate an ever-increasing frequency of hospital visits, several requiring

ambulance service. Once at the hospital we had to conform to the process—if Venesa was not admitted we would go home after picking up a prescribed medication from the pharmacy, if admitted I was prepared to stay the night with her. Flexibility was the name of the game. Pneumonia and urinary tract infections seemed to be Venesa's most frequent issues. Her most notable hospitalization was for aspiration phenomena and congestive heart failure, compounded by an acute respiratory attack while she was already hospitalized. Fortunately, I had been staying in the room with her to advocate for her and I was there when she sat up in bed at 3:00 a.m. with a distressed look, proclaiming "I can't breathe." Indeed, she was gasping for air. It was surprisingly difficult to find a nurse at that hour, but once found, the nurse called for a team of medical professionals who relieved Venesa's immediate distress by placing a pressure oxygen mask on her face. Once she was stabilized, she was relocated to the critical care unit for the remainder of her hospital stay.

One of the critical care unit doctors informed me that it was very likely that Venesa did not have aspiration pneumonia but that the problem with her lungs was probably caused by congestive heart failure.

I was dismayed to learn that we would have to make additional adjustments to Venesa's care for the balance of her life:

- All food was to be pureed, and all liquids were to be thickened to avoid possible aspiration of food into her lungs;
- Venesa was never to be allowed to get out of bed alone again—she was a fall risk;
- She would not be allowed to walk on her own or stand in the shower;
- She would require around-the-clock care;

- Venesa was put on Hospice;
- Hospice provided a hospital bed for Venesa, which we put in the family room so Venesa would not feel isolated. The bed was in place before we got home from the hospital.

Learning about the resources and provisions of Hospice was insightful. The in-home care had both positive and negative experiences. Hospice provides periodic home-care visits by a nurse, specialists to provide physical therapy, help to give sponge baths in bed, and a social worker to provide support. It also covers the cost of some medications and provides emotional support and guidance to the family and caregivers.

While initially this additional care was helpful, one day Hospice sent a substitute social worker to help. She had never met us before, knew little about Venesa, and was scarcely in the house for 5 minutes when she observed my helping Venesa to walk and heard me say, "Yesterday we took three steps; today let's try to take four steps." With that, the social worker silently left the house and reported me to Adult Protective Services for "elder abuse." The Hospice nurse who came the day after the incident told me this had been reported, and although I was not supposed to know about the charge, I was prepared when a representative from Adult Protective Services came to the house. The representative would not explain the reason for the visit. She informed me that while there was no complaint, she just came to make sure that Venesa was okay. I reported that Venesa was sleeping and that there was no reason of sufficient gravity to wake her up. Despite the woman's insistence, I suggested she go pick on someone else and firmly closed the door.

I then relieved Hospice from its service; our routine regained stability and we were much more comfortable without the questionable help. When the Hospice administration found out what had happened, the director called me into a meeting with the complete staff; we discussed the incident, they apologized to me, and reported in writing to Adult Protective Services that there had been a mistake and all was well in our household. While I still did not retain its service at that time, I know Hospice has extended invaluable help to many other families as they face the end-of life-process. In the last few days before Venesa's passing, I again relied on Hospice and benefited from its exceptional service at a time of great need.

Therapeutic Measures
We were very fortunate to have a particularly well-qualified and knowledgeable physical therapist, Debra, supporting Venesa. Debra had studied the cognitive interaction between the brain and the body as well as traditional physical therapy. Most of the physical therapy Debra assigned to Venesa focused on developing balance and maintaining muscle strength. Balance exercises included walking from her chair to the kitchen sink and standing there without support unless Venesa needed to steady herself to avoid a fall. She would practice rising to stand on her toes multiple times, then stand flat-footed on a soft mat by the sink. Holding the balanced position for several minutes, she would alternate between balancing with her eyes open and then with her eyes closed. Venesa would walk the length of the kitchen counter sideways several times, steadying herself with the counter if need be. Then Venesa would return to her chair across the room and practice getting up and sitting down numerous times to help with leg strength. A ball would be placed between Venesa's knees and she was to squeeze her knees together and release several times; then a stretch resistance band would be tied around her knees and she would be told to push her knees apart, then release and repeat several times. We walked Venesa around the house as much as she was comfortable with. Naturally Debra

explained what was going on with the cognitive interaction as the exercises were completed.

Among the most successful therapies was a balloon batting exercise designed to help with hand-to-eye coordination. Debbie and I would bat a balloon to Venesa, who was sitting in a chair and she was to volley it back to us. One day, the balloon volley went so well that we tried it with Venesa standing up. We were delighted to see how well she was able to do it, so we took an even bolder step. If she could hit a balloon standing up, would she be able to hit a ball on the tennis court? So we tried it. For safety, we put a gait belt on her and had her stand on one side of a tennis court net. I held the gait belt loosely to provide balance if she needed it and Debbie would hand feed her tennis balls from the other side of the net. Using a normal full-size tennis racket, Venesa could successfully hit up to 120 balls, stepping into each ball as appropriate (forehand or backhand) and she was able to return about 80 percent of the balls over the net. Granted, Venesa had been a very accomplished tennis player in her day, even winning the club championship. And even in dementia—with her compromised balance and mobility—she was able to thrive in the mechanics of a sport she had once enjoyed so much. I was so pleased to have envisioned the possibilities of movement rather than focusing on the limitations of the circumstances.

When I began to support and stand Venesa up with the gait belt, we were able to get her to walk again, albeit for only a few steps at a time. This made it possible for her to shower again (using her disability shower chair) and normalized her activities a little.

We undertook another very successful form of therapy in October 2015. I took Venesa to the accredited Hearts Therapeutic Equestrian Center, which focuses on enhancing the capabilities, self-esteem, and independence of special-needs children and adults through the power of horsemanship. The focus is on physical, cognitive, and/or emotional challenges due to illness, injury, age, or disability.

Evidently, the gait of the rear end of a horse is closest to the gait of the human pelvis and horseback riding stimulates the base of the spine and transmits signals to the brain, helping the cognitively impaired. Naturally, riding a horse also helps with balance and with strengthening core muscles.

The feasibility of Venesa's riding a horse was tested on a beautiful fall morning and after that first ride she was accepted into the program. She seemed to love riding her assigned horse, Sage, a large and very docile horse whose demeanor resembled that of a service dog. He seemed to understand that he was carrying very delicate cargo and acted accordingly.

The large high-backed wheelchair that Venesa was confined to initially spooked Sage, but he quickly got accustomed to it. The process of mounting Sage was to wheel Venesa up a ramp and onto a platform and bring Sage to the edge of the platform. Venesa, with the help of several attendants, would be taken up next to the saddle; she would stand up and lean against the saddle while the wheelchair was removed, and once Venesa was lifted onto the saddle she rotated 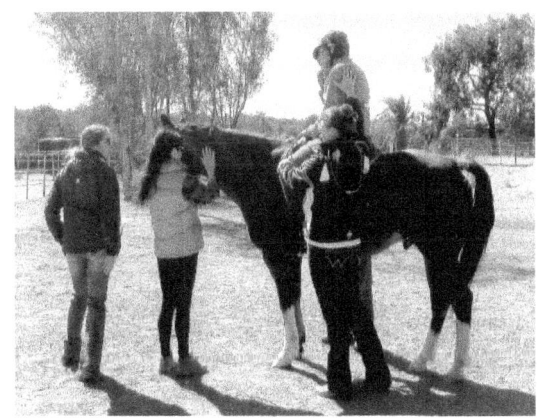 her right leg over the saddle and was in place to ride.

Two of four support personnel were positioned on either side of the horse to ensure Venesa's balance. They initially held her in place while a third person holding the reins slowly led Sage. They would gradually let go of Venesa, yet stayed in position lest Venesa were to begin to fall. She was able to ride alone for up to ten minutes at a time before she would start to fall. A fourth person, the walk leader, directed the operation and monitored Venesa's demeanor to ensure that she was okay.

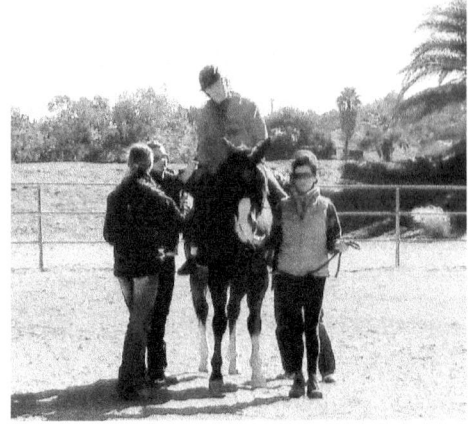

The report at the conclusion of this program stated that Venesa had a slight improvement in core/trunk strength, range of motion, balance, posture, stamina, normalization of muscle tone, and speech. Further, at a time when Venesa had essentially stopped talking, it was clear that she answered simple questions when riding Sage.

I truly wish I had tried this earlier. Not only did Venesa seem to love riding, but it proved to be an effective therapy. Unfortunately, she only had the opportunity to ride about six times, the last of which was two months to the day before her passing.

Providing some form of occupational therapy while at home was also one of my concerns. When Venesa began to lie back in her reclining chair and stare at the ceiling in 2014, I was concerned at the complete mental vacuum of her spending hours looking up at a blank ceiling. Debbie suggested that we hang an infant's mobile on the ceiling above her recliner to provide some visual stimulation. After thinking about it, we settled on tying a group of colorful and odd-shaped helium balloons around her chair. Not only were they stimulating for her to look at, but she enjoyed playing with them as well. This very simple source of stimulation turned out to be very effective in holding Venesa's attention, and providing her with entertainment. We learned that metallic foil balloons hold helium much longer than latex balloons and that they are refillable.

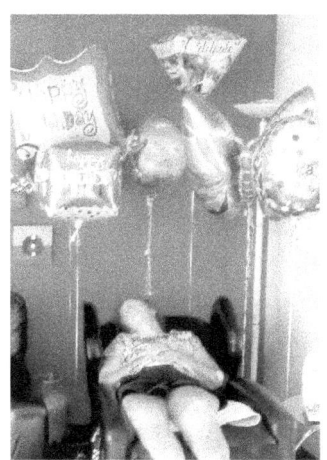

Culinary Adjustments

While in the hospital for congestive heart failure, a speech therapist had come into Venesa's room on doctors' orders to test Venesa's ability to swallow. Taking the conservative approach, the therapist had ordered Venesa's diet to be changed to pureed food and thickened liquids immediately, in a single step function, with no transition!

Charged with the responsibility of preventing aspiration of food by pureeing all solids and thickening all liquids, I realized that Venesa did not like pureed food in general, particularly not the pureed meat. I called it "mystery meat" because only the person who pureed it had any idea what it was. She did not eat well.

The opinion of the doctor in the critical care unit—that Venesa may not have had aspiration pneumonia—resonated in my mind along with Venesa's statement in her Advanced Healthcare Directive: ". . . if I am suffering from a terminal condition from which death is expected . . . . I request that all treatments other than those needed to keep me comfortable be discontinued or withheld and my physician(s) allow me to die as gently as possible."

Armed with this mindset, I decided to engage the doctor in a discussion of the right path to follow for Venesa's nutrition, while understanding the risks involved. We decided to take a very slow, gentle, conservative approach to minimize any risk and try to wean her off thickened liquids and pureed foods in an attempt to significantly increase her pleasure and quality of life.

The first step was to give Venesa plain water with no thickener. Happily, she did not aspirate the water or any of the pureed food she had with it for the first month. We then stopped thickening other liquids that accompanied her pureed foods for the next several weeks. She did not aspirate that either. We progressed to a mechanically soft diet with no thickened liquids and no pureed food; again, no aspiration occurred. It worked!

Encouraged by this, after a matter of months we transitioned Venesa back to a traditional diet, carefully cutting hard-to-chew foods such as meats and pizza into small bite-size portions. Venesa began to eat much better once she was back on a normal diet and seemed much happier. I did supplement her diet toward the end with four to six Ensure Plus beverages each day to augment meals. By doing this, she maintained her normal weight to the end. The duration of each meal required patience, taking from one to two hours; Venesa would take a bite or two, hallucinate for several minutes, then take another bite. This pattern remained constant for the remainder of her life. Venesa's hallucinations were visual, pleasant, and, although frequent, usually very short.

Approaching Venesa's Final Days

Christmas 2015 was a time of very high highs and very low lows. A close friend, Sandra, had suggested that I take Venesa out for a festive Christmas dinner. I thought the stimulation of the fancy restaurant, with its lavish, over-the-top, festive Christmas decorations, would bring Venesa joy—which it did. While we were waiting to be seated, Sandra briefly stopped in to wish us a Merry Christmas. Venesa, clearly recognizing her, also said "Merry Christmas," smiling broadly, reaching out to greet Sandra. A festive tone was well established.

Venesa had a great time; she ate all of her huge prime rib dinner with all the fixings. I had cut up her meat and, for the most part, she was successful in feeding herself and then went on to dessert. Albeit non-verbally, she interacted with the service personnel, and seemed to enjoy herself. However, by the time we got home, the festive mood was broken. Venesa had no interest in opening her Christmas presents—in fact, I do not believe she even knew what they were.

We spent the day after Christmas at home. Debbie and I encouraged her to open her presents, but she was unable to unwrap them, not even with our help. After such a happy Christmas day, it was simply a low day for her. Even when we opened the gifts for her, she had little reaction.

Venesa and I saw 2016 in with a quiet evening at home.

In late January 2016 I took Venesa to the hospital emergency room because she was very lethargic and had labored breathing. She was admitted to the hospital, and after extensive testing, it was noted that the size of her brain was shrinking and she was diagnosed with a severe blood infection. The bacteria was believed to have been introduced by an infection related to a foreign object in her body (perhaps her pacemaker, a pacemaker wire, or one of her two knee replacements). Venesa remained in the hospital for a full week as testing continued; she was not responding to the prescribed intravenous antibiotic, described by the doctor as the "biggest tool in the toolbox." This antibiotic was to be administered for six weeks, with the dose modified each week based on results of the weekly blood tests. I was warned that if this did not work, it could very well be Venesa's demise. Once all testing was completed, the doctor recommended that I take her home—keeping Venesa in the hospital posed the risk of exposing her to other germs and diseases unnecessarily. So I took her home and continued to give her the daily intravenous antibiotics for four and a half weeks.

After returning to our home routine, Venesa seemed to need more sleep than she had before. The infection had taken its toll. However, with the Hoyer lift, the wheelchair, and wheelchair van we were out and about for walks in the park and the neighborhood and running errands. She was eating, drinking her Ensure Plus, regaining some strength, but all activity was at a slower pace.

In early March, Debbie advised me that she suspected that the strange low noises Venesa was making and her subdued demeanor might be an indication that she was in pain and needed a stronger medication for pain. By then, Venesa herself was unable to talk so she could not tell us.

Consulting with Venesa's primary care physician about this resulted in replacing her pain medication with an extremely small dose of morphine. Wow! What a difference that made! She seemed so relaxed, calm, and comfortable. I had had no idea that she might have been uncomfortable.

At this point I called our sons, Jeff and Chad, and told them that their mother was beginning to fail. Jeff came immediately to stay with his mom and support me. Chad, however, was on government business in Tokyo, and it would take a few days to get authorization to return to the United States.

Since it was evident that Chad might not make it home before Venesa passed, Jeff suggested that we should set up a time for a Skype video conference for Chad and his mother. Putting a computer where Venesa could see it and hear Chad's voice, Jeff initiated the call and left the room, giving Chad some private time with his mother. They visited this way for well over an hour. As it turned out, Chad was not able to return before Venesa passed, so it was fortunate that they had had that time together.

Jeff also spent time alone with his mother, talking to her and reminiscing over fond memories they had shared. Throughout the afternoon, Jeff played Venesa's favorite Broadway show scores. Although Venesa was not able to talk, her body language indicated her pleasure in the time they spent together.

Venesa was confined to her bed for her final day and a half. It was too painful for her to be moved so I kept her comfortable in bed with morphine every two hours for her final two days, and by now, she was back under Hospice care. Jeff took the midnight shift on March 11, and administered Venesa's morphine. With such deep relaxation, Jeff thought he had lost her and ran to alert me. But she had waited for me to join her in our bedroom and we were able to say our final goodbye. I gave her a hug and a kiss and told her how much I loved her. She took two breaths, mustered up the energy to say "good bye, ok," took one more breath, and passed into Heaven.

Venesa's Legacy

Venesa loved teaching, the Academy of Nutrition and Dietetics, and the Registered Dietitian profession. To honor her lifelong interests, I initiated a perpetual National Scholarship through the Academy of Nutrition and Dietetics Foundation, which is available to students interested in the Registered Dietitian Certification. The scholarship is known as The Venesa W. Strong RD, MNS, MBA Memorial Scholarship. The first scholarship is to be awarded in October 2017.

www.ingramcontent.com/pod-product-compliance
Lightning Source LLC
Chambersburg PA
CBHW070316230526
45470CB00002B/899